The Healthy Mediterranean Way of Eating

Balance your lifestyle with energetic tasteful recipes

Lana Green

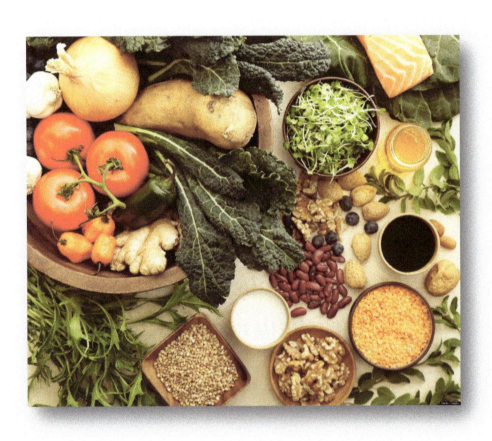

© copyright 2021 – all rights reserved.

the content contained within this book may not be reproduced, duplicated or transmitted without direct written permission from the author or the publisher.

under no circumstances will any blame or legal responsibility be held against the publisher, or author, for any damages, reparation, or monetary loss due to the information contained within this book. either directly or indirectly.

legal notice:

this book is copyright protected. this book is only for personal use. you cannot amend, distribute, sell, use, quote or paraphrase any part, or the content within this book, without the consent of the author or publisher.

disclaimer notice:

please note the information contained within this document is for educational and entertainment purposes only. all effort has been executed to present accurate, up to date, and reliable, complete information. no warranties of any kind are declared or implied. readers acknowledge that the author is not engaging in the rendering of legal, financial, medical or professional advice. the content within this book has been derived from various sources. please consult a licensed professional before attempting any techniques outlined in this book.

by reading this document, the reader agrees that under no circumstances is the author responsible for any losses, direct or indirect, which are incurred as a result of the use of information contained within this document, including, but not limited to, — errors, omissions, or inaccuracies.

Table of Contents

- CAULIFLOWER FRITTERS 6
- MEDITERRANEAN CHICKPEA SNACK 9
- AVOCADO CHICKPEA PIZZA 11
- PITA WEDGES WITH ALMOND BEAN DIP 13
- GINGER ANTIPASTI 15
- MEDITERRANEAN CHICKPEA SPREAD 17
- ROSEMARY BEETS 19
- SCALLIONS DIP 21
- DILL TAPAS 23
- SOUR CREAM DIP 24
- ARUGULA ANTIPASTI 26
- GOAT CHEESE DIP 28
- MOZZARELLA DIP 30
- SPICY SALSA 32
- CHEESE SPREAD 34
- PROSCIUTTO BEANS 36
- CARROT CHIPS 37
- ANTIPASTI SALAD 39
- BLACK OLIVES SPREAD 40
- BELL PEPPER ANTIPASTI 42
- HUMMUS RINGS 44
- FISH STRIPS 45
- VEGETABLE BALLS 47
- ITALIAN STYLE EGGPLANT CHIPS 49
- LENTIL DIP 51
- OVERNIGHT OATS 53
- MJADERA 55
- BANANA CHEESECAKE CHOCOLATE COOKIES 57
- CHEESECAKE ICE CREAM 59
- VANILLA CUSTARD 61
- CHOCOLATE CHEESECAKE SHAKE 63

- PISTACHIO MILK-SHAKE 64
- CHOCOLATE CRUNCH COOKIES 66
- CANDIED CORN PUFFS 68
- CUCUMBER AND RANCH DRESSING 70
- BAKED CHEESE CRISP 72
- CAULIFLOWER BREADSTICKS 73
- STRAWBERRY VINAIGRETTE 75
- ASIAN CHICKEN SALAD WRAPS 77
- GREEN-BERRY SMOOTHIE 79
- MATCHA GREEN TEA SMOOTHIE 81
- BLUEBERRY AND COCONUT SMOOTHIE 83
- POMEGRANATE SMOOTHIE WITH CRANBERRIES 85
- PASTA SALAD ISRAELI 88
- AMAZING CAULIFLOWER PIZZA 91
- FLATBREADS MEDITERRANEAN 96
- SPINACH FETA GRILLED CHEESE 99
- HUMMUS 102
- BABA GANOUSH(VEGAN) 104
- SPICED ALMONDS 106

Cauliflower Fritters

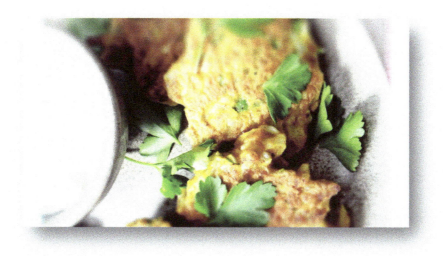

Prep Time: 10 min

Cook Time: 50 min

Serve: 4

Ingredients:

- 30 oz. canned chickpeas, drained and rinsed
- 2 and ½ tbsp. olive oil
- 1 small yellow onion, chopped

- 2 cups cauliflower florets chopped
- 2 tbsp. garlic, minced
- A pinch of salt and black pepper

Preparation:

1. Spread half of the chickpeas on a baking sheet lined with parchment pepper, add 1 tbsp. oil, season with salt and pepper, toss and bake at 400°F for 30 minutes.

2. Transfer the chickpeas to a food processor, pulse well and put the mix into a bowl.

3. Heat a pan with the ½ tbsp. oil over medium-high heat, add the garlic and the onion and sauté for 3 minutes.

4. Add the cauliflower, cook for 6 minutes more, transfer this to a blender, add the rest of the chickpeas,

pulse, pour over the crispy chickpeas mix from the bowl, stir and shape medium patties out of this mix. Heat a pan with the rest of the oil over medium-high heat, add the patties, cook them for 3 minutes on each side, and serve breakfast.

Mediterranean Chickpea Snack

Prep Time: 30 min

Cook Time: 0 min

Serve: 2

Ingredients:

- ½ tsp. garlic powder
- 1 can (10 oz.) chickpeas, rinsed and drained
- ½ tsp. dried basil
- 1 tsp. extra-virgin olive oil
- ¼ tsp. sea salt
- 1 tsp. Nutritional Yeast
- ¼ tsp. red pepper flakes

Preparation:

1. Preheat the oven to 450°F. Line a baking pan with a parchment paper. Grease it with some refined coconut oil or avocado oil (You can also use cooking spray). Combine the chickpeas, seasonings, and oil in a mixing bowl.

2. Arrange the chickpeas in the pan. Roast the chickpeas for about 10 minutes. Toss and keep roasting for 10 more minutes. Serve warm.

Avocado Chickpea Pizza

Prep Time: 20 min

Cook Time: 20 min

Serve: 2

Ingredients:

- 1 and ¼ cups chickpea flour
- A pinch of salt and black pepper
- 1 and ¼ cups water
- 2 tbsp. olive oil
- 1 tsp. onion powder
- 1 tsp. garlic, minced
- 1 tomato, sliced
- 1 avocado, peeled, pitted and sliced
- 2 oz. gouda, sliced

- ¼ cup tomato sauce
- 2 tbsp. green onions, chopped

Preparation:

1. In a bowl, mix the chickpea flour with salt, pepper, water, the oil, onion powder and the garlic, stir well until you obtain a dough, knead a bit, put in a bowl, cover and leave aside for 20 minutes. Transfer the dough to a working surface, shape a bit circle, transfer it to a baking sheet lined with parchment paper and bake at 425°F for 10 minutes.

2. Spread the tomato sauce over the pizza, spread the rest of the ingredients and bake at 400°F for 10 minutes more.

3. Cut and serve for breakfast.

Pita Wedges with Almond Bean Dip

Prep Time: 10 min

Cook Time: 5 min

Serve: 5

Ingredients:

- 8 oz. beet, cubed
- 5 garlic cloves, peeled
- ¼ cup almond, slivered
- 15 ½ oz. garbanzo beans
- ¾ cup extra-virgin olive oil
- 1 ½ tbsp. red wine vinegar
- Whole-wheat pita wedges to serve

Preparation:

1. In a saucepan or deep skillet, boil the beet in sufficient water quantity until it is tender. Drain, peel, cut in cubes and blend in a food processor. Add the garbanzo beans, almonds, oil, and garlic and blend everything well until smooth. Add the red wine and blend for one more minute.

2. Season with black pepper and salt.

3. Chill in the refrigerator. Serve with pita wedges.

Ginger Antipasti

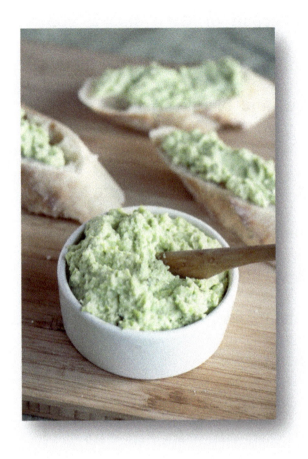

Prep Time: 10 min

Cook Time: 0 min

Serve: 6

Ingredients:

- 1 tsp. ginger powder
- 1 cup fresh parsley, chopped
- 1 tbsp. apple cider vinegar
- 3 tbsp. avocado oil
- 2 oz celery stalk, chopped

Preparation:

Mix all ingredients in the bowl and leave for 5 minutes in the fridge.

Mediterranean Chickpea Spread

Prep Time: 8 min

Cook Time: 5 min

Serve: 2

Ingredients:

- 2 cups chickpeas (canned or pre-soaked and cooked)
- 2 tbsp. lemon juice
- 1/2 tsp. cumin
- 2 cloves garlic, minced
- 4 tsp. olive oil
- Salt to taste
- Ground cinnamon (optional)

Preparation:

1. In a mixing bowl, add the chickpeas; mash thoroughly using a fork (you can also use a blender).

2. Add the olive oil, garlic and lemon juice. Combine well; top with some cinnamon. Serve with vegetable sticks, whole-wheat crackers, or whole-wheat pita wedges.

Rosemary Beets

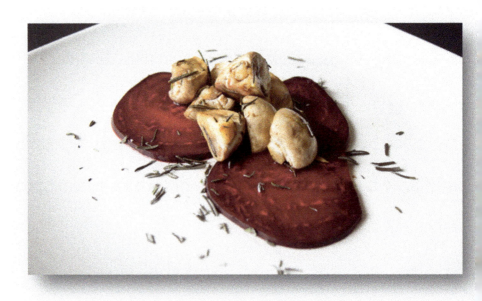

Prep Time: 10 min

Cook Time: 4 min

Serve: 6

Ingredients:

- 1-lb. beets, sliced, peeled
- 2 tbsp. lemon juice
- 1 tsp. dried rosemary

- ¼ tsp. garlic powder
- 1 tbsp. olive oil

Preparation:

Sprinkle the beets with lemon juice, rosemary, garlic powder, and olive oil. Then preheat the grill to 400°F. Place the sliced beet in the grill and cook it for 2 minutes per side.

Scallions Dip

Prep Time: 5 min

Cook Time: 15 min

Serve: 4

Ingredients:

- 1 cup spinach, chopped
- 2 oz scallions, chopped
- ¼ cup plain yogurt
- ¼ tsp. chili powder
- 1 tsp. olive oil

Preparation:

1. Melt the olive oil in the saucepan. Add spinach and scallions. Saute the greens for 10 minutes.

2. Then add chili powder and plain yogurt. Stir well and cook it for 5 minutes more. Then blend the mixture with the help of the immersion blender.

Dill Tapas

Prep Time: 5 min

Cook Time: 0 min

Serve: 8

Ingredients:

- ½ tsp. garlic powder
- 2 cups plain yogurt
- ½ cup dill, chopped
- ¼ tsp. ground black pepper
- 2 pecans, chopped
- 2 tbsp. lemon juice

Preparation:

Put all ingredients in the bowl and stir well with the help of the spoon.

Sour Cream Dip

Prep Time: 10 min

Cook Time: 0 min

Serve: 8

Ingredients:

- 4 oz yogurt
- ¼ tsp. chili flakes
- ¼ tsp. salt
- 2 avocados, peeled, pitted
- 1 tsp. olive oil
- ½ tsp. lemon juice
- 2 tbsp. fresh parsley, chopped

Preparation:

1. Put all ingredients in the blender and blend until smooth.

2. Store the dip in the closed vessel in the fridge for up to 5 days.

Arugula Antipasti

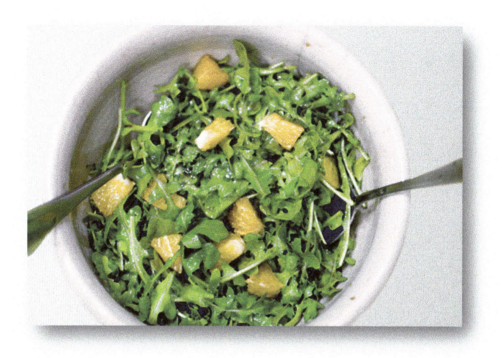

Prep Time: 5 min

Cook Time: 0 min

Serve: 8

Ingredients:

- 2 oz chives, chopped
- 1 cup arugula, chopped
- 2 cups chickpeas, canned
- 1 jalapeno pepper, chopped
- 1 tbsp. avocado oil
- 1 tsp. lemon juice

Preparation:

Put all ingredients in the bowl and stir well.

Goat Cheese Dip

Prep Time: 10 min

Cook Time: 8 min

Serve: 4

Ingredients:

- 3 oz goats cheese, soft
- 2 oz plain yogurt
- 2 oz chives, chopped
- 1 tbsp. lemon juice
- ¼ tsp. ground black pepper
- 2 bell peppers

Preparation:

1. Grill the bell peppers for 3-4 minutes per side.

2. Then peel the peppers and remove seeds.

3. Then put bell peppers in the blender. Add all remaining ingredients, blend them well and transfer in the ramekins.

Mozzarella Dip

Prep Time: 10 min

Cook Time: 20 min

Serve: 10

Ingredients:

- 1-lb. artichoke hearts, diced
- ¾ cup spinach, chopped
- 1 cup mozzarella cheese, grated
- 1 tsp. Italian seasonings
- ½ tsp. garlic powder
- ¼ cup organic almond milk

Preparation:

Put all ingredients in the saucepan, stir well, and close the lid. Saute the meal on low heat for 20 minutes. Stir it from time to time. Then chill the dip well.

Spicy Salsa

Prep Time: 40 min

Cook Time: 0 min

Serve: 16

Ingredients:

- 3 cups tomatoes, chopped
- 1 tsp. salt
- 1 tsp. white pepper
- ½ cup red onion, chopped
- 1 cup fresh cilantro, chopped
- 1 jalapeno pepper, chopped 1 tbsp. olive oil
- 1 tbsp. apple cider vinegar

Preparation:

1. Put all ingredients in the salad bowl and mix well.

2. Leave the cooked salsa for 30 minutes in the fridge.

Cheese Spread

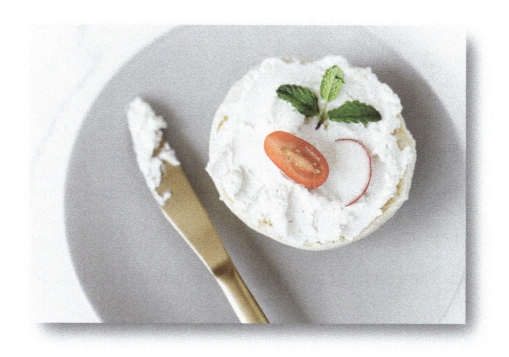

Prep Time: 10 min

Cook Time: 8 min

Serve: 6

Ingredients:

- ½ cup cream cheese

- 1 pickle, grated
- 1 oz fresh dill, chopped
- ¼ tsp. ground paprika

Preparation:

1. Carefully mix cream cheese with dill and ground paprika.

2. Then add a grated pickle and gently mix the spread.

Prosciutto Beans

Prep Time: 10 min

Cook Time: 0 min

Serve: 8

Ingredients:

- 2 cups canned cannellini beans, drained
- 1 tbsp. scallions, diced
- 3 tbsp. olive oil
- ¼ tsp. chili flakes 1 tbsp. lemon juice
- 3 oz beef, chopped, cooked

Preparation:

Put all ingredients in the bowl and stir well.

Carrot Chips

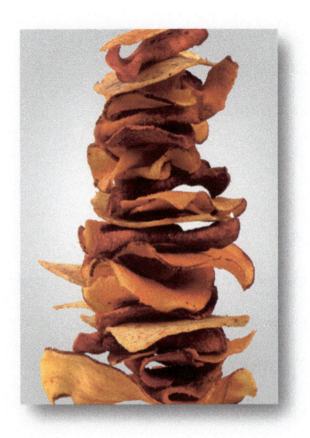

Prep Time: 5 min

Cook Time: 10 min

Serve: 6

Ingredients:

- 2 carrots, thinly sliced
- 1 tsp. salt
- 1 tsp. olive oil

Preparation:

1. Line the baking tray with baking paper. Then arrange the sliced carrot in one layer.

2. Sprinkle the vegetables with olive oil and salt. Bake the carrot chips for 10 minutes or until the vegetables are crunchy.

Antipasti Salad

Prep Time: 10 min

Cook Time: 0 min

Serve: 4

Ingredients:

- ½ cup green olives, pitted and sliced
- 1 cucumber, spiralized
- 1 cup cherry tomatoes, halved
- 4 oz Feta cheese, crumbled
- 2 tbsp. olive oil

Preparation:

1. Put green olives, spiralized cucumber, and cherry tomatoes in the bowl. Add olive oil and stir well.

2. Then top the salad with Feta.

Black Olives Spread

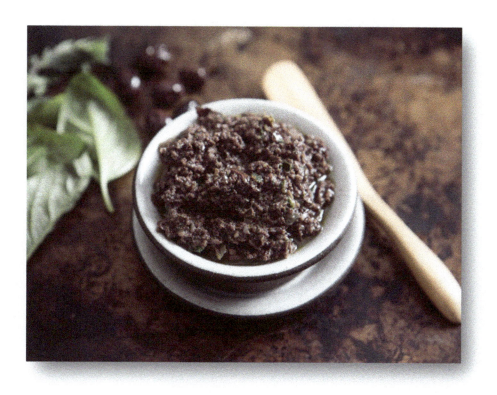

Prep Time: 10 min

Cook Time: 0 min

Serve: 10

Ingredients:

- 3 cups black olives, pitted
- ½ cup chickpeas, canned
- 1 tsp. Italian seasonings
- 3 tbsp. sunflower oil
- ½ tsp. ground black pepper

Preparation:

Put all ingredients in the blender and blend until smooth.

Bell Pepper Antipasti

Prep Time: 10 min

Cook Time: 4 min

Serve: 6

Ingredients:

- 5 bell peppers
- 1 tbsp. olive oil
- 3 tbsp. avocado oil
- ½ tsp. salt
- 2 garlic cloves, minced
- 3 tbsp. fresh cilantro, chopped

Preparation:

1. Pierce the bell peppers with the help of a knife and sprinkle with olive oil. Grill the vegetables at 400F for 2 minutes per side. Then peel them and remove seeds.

2. Put the grilled bell peppers in the blender and add all remaining ingredients. Blend the mixture well.

Hummus Rings

Prep Time: 10 min

Cook Time: 0 min

Serve: 4

Ingredients:

- ½ cup hummus
- 2 cucumbers

Preparation:

Roughly slice the cucumbers and remove the cucumber flesh. Then fill every cucumber ring with hummus.

Fish Strips

Prep Time: 10 min

Cook Time: 0 min

Serve: 4

Ingredients:

- 1 cucumber, sliced
- 1 tsp. apple cider vinegar
- 2 tbsp. plain yogurt
- 1 tsp. dried dill
- 3 oz salmon, smoked, sliced

Preparation:

1. Arrange the sliced cucumber in the plate in one layer.

2. Then sprinkle them with apple cider vinegar, plain yogurt, and dried dill.

3. Then top the cucumbers with sliced salmon.

Vegetable Balls

Prep Time: 10 min

Cook Time: 5 min

Serve: 8

Ingredients:

- 2 eggplants, grilled
- 2 tbsp. olive oil
- 1 garlic clove, minced
- 1 egg, beaten
- ½ cup oatmeal, ground
- ½ tsp. ground black pepper
- 2 oz Parmesan, grated

Preparation:

1. Blend the eggplants until smooth.

2. Then mix up blended eggplants with garlic, egg, oatmeal, ground black pepper, and Parmesan. Make the small balls.

3. Heat the skillet with olive oil and put the eggplant balls inside. Roast them for on high heat for 1 minute per side.

Italian Style Eggplant Chips

Prep Time: 10 min

Cook Time: 5 min

Serve: 10

Ingredients:

- 2 eggplants, thinly sliced
- 1 tsp. ground black pepper
- 1 tsp. Italian seasonings
- 1 tbsp. olive oil

Preparation:

1. Rub the eggplant sliced with ground black pepper and Italian seasonings.

2. Then sprinkle the vegetable sliced with olive oil.

3. Grill the eggplant sliced for 2 minutes per side at 400F or until the vegetables are crunchy.

Lentil Dip

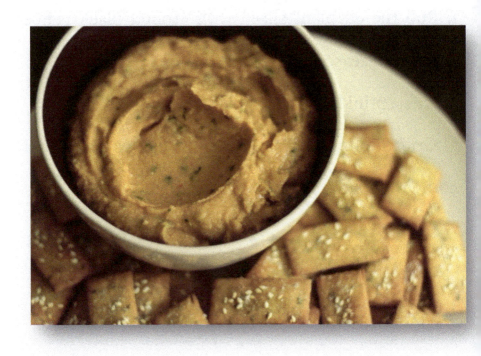

Prep Time: 10 min

Cook Time: 0 min

Serve: 7

Ingredients:

- 1 cup green lentils, cooked

- 1 tbsp. apple cider vinegar
- 1 tomato, chopped
- 1 tsp. olive oil
- 2 oz Parmesan, grated

Preparation:

Mix up all ingredients in the bowl and blend gently with the help of the immersion blender.

Overnight Oats

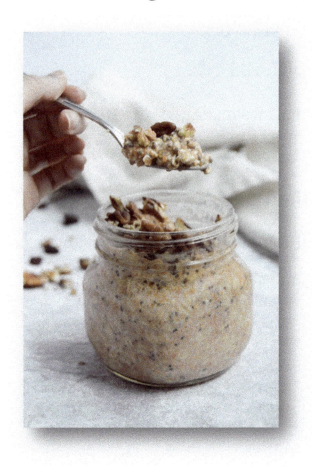

Prep Time: 7 min

Cook Time: 0 min

Serve: 2

Ingredients:

- 1.5 cups Rolled Oats
- 1 cup Tinned coconut milk
- 1.5 cup Almond Milk
- 2 tbsp Chia Seeds
- ½ tsp Ground Cinnamon

Preparation:

Blend all the ingredients.

Mjadera

Prep Time: 7 min

Cook Time: 0 min

Serve: 4

Ingredients:

- 1 Cup Brown lentils
- 1 cup Bulgur
- One Chopped Onion
- 2 tbsp Avocado or grapeseed oil
- 1/4 cup olive oil
- Salt

Preparation:

1. Wash lentils & crook in the pot along with three cups water on moderate heat for fifteen minutes. Lentils should be dente.

2. When lentils are cooking, cut the onion into dices and sauté with cooking oil and sauté and oil in a pan till brown. The darker the onion, is more flavorful the dish will be.

3. Add uncooked bulgur, caramelized onion, one-fourth cup of olive oil, 1 cup water & salt according to taste. These are added into semi- cooked lentils on moderate heat till they are cooked fully.

4. If the water dries and still lentils aren't cooked properly, add water according to need and cook again.

Banana Cheesecake Chocolate Cookies

Prep Time: 20 min

Cook Time: 25 min

Serve: 14

Ingredients:

- Crust
- 2 tbsp butter
- 12 cookies Oreo Cheesecakes
- 1 tsp vanilla extract
- 2 tbsp flour
- 1/4 cup cream
- 1/2 cup sugar
- 1/2 cup chocolate chips

- 2 * 8 oz. cream cheese 1/2 cup banana
- One egg
- Chocolate Whipped Cream
- 1 cup heavy whipping cream
- 1/4 cup cocoa powder
- 2 Tablespoons mini chocolate chips
- 1/2 cup powdered sugar
- 1/2 teaspoon rum extract
- One yellow banana, sliced

Preparation:

1. Blend all the mixture in the blender except eggs and banana. Now whisk egg and banana and make a batter.

2. Bake the batter in the oven at 350 degrees for twenty-five minutes. Top the cookies with cocoa, cream, vanilla, and sugar mixture. Serve and enjoy.

Cheesecake Ice Cream

Prep Time: 20 min

Cook Time: 20 min

Serve: 1.5 quarts

Ingredients:

- 1 cup milk
- Two eggs
- 2.5 cups cream
- 1 tsp vanilla extract
- 1-1/4 cups sugar
- 12 oz. cream cheese
- 1 tbsp lemon juice

Preparation:

1. Melt sugar in cream and milk mixture. Whisk in egg and transfer in a pan. Cook over medium flame.

2. Remove from flame and mix in cream cheese. Cool the mixture and stir in lemon juice and vanilla extract.

3. Refrigerate it for 120 minutes and serve.

Vanilla Custard

Prep Time: 10 min

Cook Time: 20 min

Serve: 4

Ingredients:

- 1 tbsp corn-flour
- 1/3 cup sugar
- 1 Vanilla Bean
- 1 cup milk
- Four yolks of egg
- 1 cup cream

Preparation:

1. Cook vanilla, milk, and cream in a saucepan with continuous stirring. Pour cream mixture over egg, sugar, and corn flour mixture in a bowl.

2. Cook until the required thickness is achieved.

3. Cook and serve.

Chocolate Cheesecake Shake

Prep Time: 10 min

Cook Time: 0 min

Serve: 4

Ingredients:

Six scoops of ice cream (chocolate flavor)

oz. cream cheese

2 cups of milk

Preparation:

1. Blend milk and cream cheese in a food processor.

2. Transfer the mixture to a serving glass and add ice cream and serve.

Pistachio Milk-Shake

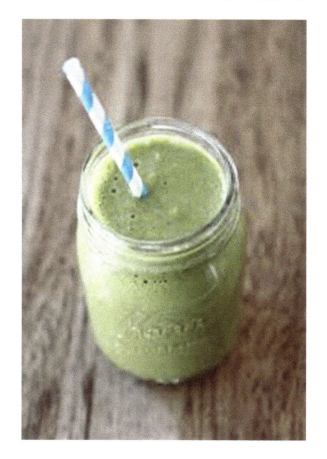

Prep Time: 5 min

Cook Time: 0 min

Serve: 4 glasses

Ingredients:

1 tsp vanilla extract

- 4 tbsp pistachios
- 5 cups ice cream (pistachio)
- Pinch of salt
- 1 cup milk

Preparation:

Mix all the ingredients in a blender and serve.

Chocolate Crunch Cookies

Prep Time: 15 min

Cook Time: 10 min

Serve: 35

Ingredients:

- 1/2 cups chocolate chips
- 1.5 cups butter
- Two eggs
- One tsp baking soda
- 2 cups of sugar
- One tsp vanilla
- One tsp salt
- 1/2 cup pecans
- 2 cups oats

- 2 cups flour
- 2 cups Krispies Rice

Preparation:

1. Whisk all the ingredients in a large mixing bowl and pour the batter into a baking tray.

2. Bake in a preheated oven at 350 degrees for ten minutes.

Candied Corn Puffs

Prep Time: 15 min

Cook Time: 35 min

Serve: 8

Ingredients:

- 8 oz corn puffs
- 1 cup butter
- Salt as required
- 1 tsp baking soda
- 1 cup peanuts
- 1 cup of sugar
- 1.2 cup of corn syrup

Preparation:

1. Boil syrup, butter, and sugar. Add baking soda and transfer the mixture to a bowl with corn and peanuts.

2. Bake for 35 minutes in the oven at 250 degrees.

Cucumber and Ranch Dressing

Prep Time: 5 min

Cook Time: 0 min

Serve: 4

Ingredients:

- ½ chopped onion
- ¼ tsp pepper and salt each
- Two sliced cucumbers
- ½ tsp dill
- ½ cup ranch dressing

Preparation:

Whisk all the ingredients in a large bowl and set aside.

Serve for 40 minutes.

Baked cheese crisp

Prep Time: 5 m in

Cook Time: 8 min

Serve: 4

Ingredients:

- ¾ cup shredded cheddar
- ¾ cup parmesan cheese
- 1 tsp Italian seasoning

Preparation:

1. Mix cheese and place on a baking tray.
2. Bake for eight minutes in the oven at 400 degrees.

Cauliflower Breadsticks

Prep Time: 7 min

Cook Time: 30 min

Serve: 12

Ingredients:

- 4 lb cauliflower
- Two egg whites
- 1.5 cup Mozzarella cheese shredded
- Italian seasoning 1 tsp
- Pinch of salt
- 1/4 tsp black pepper
- Marinara sauce for dipping
- Cooking spray

Preparation:

1. Toast blended cauliflower in oven at 375 degrees for 20 minutes. Mix roasted cauliflower with egg whites, cheese, herbs, salt, pepper in a bowl.

2. Bake the mixture in the oven at 450 degrees for 18 minutes. Bring in sticks, shape, and serve.

Strawberry Vinaigrette

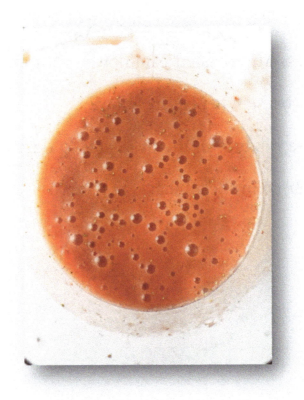

Prep Time: 10 min

Cook Time: 0 min

Serve: 9

Ingredients:

- 8 oz strawberries
- Salt to taste
- 2 tbsp apple cider vinegar
- 2 tbsp honey
- 2 tbsp olive oil
- ¼ tsp black pepper

Preparation:

Blend all the ingredients in a blender and pour in the serving dish.

Asian Chicken Salad Wraps

Prep Time: 20 min

Cook Time: 0 min

Serve: 6

Ingredients:

- 3 cup cooked chicken breasts-shredded
- 1/2 cup shredded carrot
- ¾ tsp minced gingerroot
- 3 tbsp seasoned rice vinegar
- 3 tbsp canola oil
- 2 tbsp honey
- 1 cup shredded cabbage
- 1 tbsp water
- One chopped garlic clove

- ¼ tsp pepper
- Four chopped green onions
- 1 cup cilantro leaves
- Six lettuce leaves
- Six whole-wheat tortillas

Preparation:

Whisk all the ingredients in a large mixing bowl and set aside. Place lettuce on each tortilla and spread the chicken mixture, and fold and serve.

Green-Berry Smoothie

Prep Time: 20 min

Cook Time: 0 min

Serve: 2

Ingredients:

- 1 ripe banana
- ½ cup blackcurrants take off stems baby kale leaves take off stems
- 1 cup freshly made green tea
- tsp. honey
- ice cubes

Preparation:

Dissolve the honey in the tea before you relax it. Cool first, and then blend all ingredients blender until smooth.

Matcha Green Tea Smoothie

Prep Time: 10 min

Cook Time: 0 min

Serve: 2

Ingredients:

- bananas
- tsp. Matcha green tea powder
- 1/2 tsp. vanilla bean paste or scraped from a vanilla bean pod
- 1 ½ cups milk
- 4-5 ice cubes
- tsp. honey

Preparation:

Add all ingredients except the Matcha to a blender. Blend until smooth. Sprinkle in the Matcha tea powder, stir well or blend a few seconds more or add cooled green tea).

Blueberry and Coconut Smoothie

Prep Time: 10 min

Cook Time: 0 min

Serve: 2

Ingredients:

- Portions 1 banana
- dried dates (pitted)
- 1 tsp. coconut oil
- 150g blueberries
- 300ml almond drink (almond milk)
- 1 pinch cinnamon
- tsp. grated coconut sheets fresh mint

Preparation:

1. Peel the banana and cut it into pieces. Halve dates.

2. Put coconut oil with banana, dates, blueberries, almond milk, cinnamon, and grated coconut in a blender and puree everything at the highest level until the desired consistency is achieved.

3. Fill the blueberry-coconut smoothie into 2 glasses and garnish with grated coconut and mint.

Pomegranate Smoothie with Cranberries

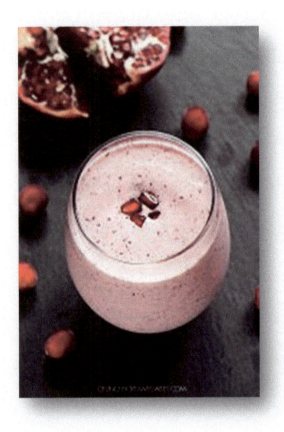

Prep Time: 20 min

Cook Time: 15 min

Serve: 2

Ingredients:

- 1 pomegranate
- 100g cranberries
- 150g yogurt (1.5% fat)
- Liquid sweetener at will 250ml milk (1.5% fat)
- Ice cubes

Preparation:

1. Cut out a wedge-shaped piece at the base of the pomegranate. Then break the fruit apart with a little pressure over a bowl so that most of the seeds fall out. Possibly work with thin rubber or disposable gloves: The juice stains strongly.

2. Set aside about 1 tbsp. of the pomegranate seeds.

3. Place the rest with the cranberries and yogurt in a tall container and finely puree with a hand blender. Season to taste with a little sweetener, add the milk and ice cubes, and mix again briefly.

4. Fill in 2 glasses and garnish with the remaining pomegranate seeds.

Pasta Salad Israeli

Prep Time: 2 h 10 min

Cook Time: 10 min

Serve: 8

Ingredients:

- 1/3 cup cucumber finely diced
- 1/3 cup radish diced
- 1/3 cup crumbled feta cheese
- 1/2 pound small pasta
- 1/3 cup tomato diced
- 1/3 cup yellow bell pepper diced
- 1/3 cup orange bell pepper diced
- 1/3 cup pepperoncini diced
- 1/3 cup black olives diced

- 1/3 cup green olives halved
- 1/3 cup red onion diced
- 1 tsp dried oregano
- 1/2 cup fresh thyme leaves
- 1 lemon juiced
- 1/4 cup olive oil more needed later on
- 1/2 tsp ground black pepper
- 1 tsp salt

Preparation:

1. Place a saucepan over medium-high heat. Fill with salted water half full. Bring to boil and add your pasta. Cook this for 10 minutes until tender. After drain and rinse in cold water.

2. Transfer your pasta to a bowl add some oil and toss until fully incorporated. Add all the remaining Ingredients: left leave the feta cheese until the end and stir well until all is mixed together.

3. Fold in cheese and refrigerate this for 2 hours. When ready to serve top the pasta salad with thyme leaves.

Amazing Cauliflower Pizza

Prep cook Time: 1 h 40 min

Serve: 4

Ingredients:

For the cauliflower crust:

- 1 1/3 cup and 4 tablespoon of grated parmesan cheese divided
- 3 pounds of cauliflower cut into small florets
- 1 tablespoon and 1 teaspoon of minced garlic
- 2 egg whites
- 1 teaspoon Italian seasoning
- 1/4 teaspoon of ground black pepper
- 1/2 teaspoon of salt
- For the Greek Yogurt Basil Sauce:
- 1/2 cup Greek yoghurt

- 1/2 cup of fresh basil chopped
- 2 teaspoon of minced garlic
- 1 tablespoon of olive oil
- 1/2 teaspoon of salt
- 1/2 teaspoon of ground black pepper

For the topping:

- 1/2 cup of parmesan cheese grated
- Roma tomatoes 3 inch 1/2 thick sliced
- 1 small Zucchini sliced
- Fresh basil for garnish
- 1/2 tablespoon of olive oil
- 1/2 teaspoon salt
- 1/2 teaspoon of ground black pepper

Preparation:

1. Preheat the oven to 400 degrees F. Meanwhile place a pizza pan with parchment sheet and set it aside.

2. Next prepare the crust for this place your cauliflower florets in a food processor and pulse in batches for 1 minute until the mixture represents rice.

3. Pour riced cauliflower in a large heat proof bowl microwave that for 14 minutes make sure to stir halfway through. Let the riced cauliflower stand for 15 minutes or until it is slightly cooked then wrap it into a thin towel and make sure a to twist to remove any excess moisture.

4. After that return the cauliflower into the bowl and add your black pepper salt garlic Italian seasoning and 1 1/3 cup cheese. Stir well until all have combined. Add your egg whites and mix well until incorporated. Divide the mixture into 2 balls each about 1 cup.

5. Then place onto prepared pizza pan and spread them evenly to form a nice crust and leave the ridge. Place your pizza pan into the oven and bake for 30 minutes until nicely golden brown.

6. While that is baking prepare for your yoghurt basil sauce. For this blend yoghurt garlic and basil until it is creamy.

7. Blend in olive oil until it is well mixed then tip the sauce in a ball and set aside until it is needed. Now prepare the topping set grill and let preheat at medium high.

8. Place your Zucchini slices in a bowl add tomatoes and your olive oil and then season nicely with pepper and salt and toss until well coated.

9. Put these vegetables on a grill rack and cook to 3 minutes per side. After it is done transfer the vegetable to a plate and set aside. Keep the grill on. When the

pizza crust is cooked remove from the oven, switch on the broiler and preheat at high for 3 minutes.

10. Put 4 remains of cheese tablespoons onto the pizza crust and then place under the broiler and cook for 2 minutes until the cheese is nicely melted and brown.

11. Remove the pizza pan from oven spread yoghurt sauce on the crust and top with your grilled vegetables and cover with remaining cheese.

12. Place the pizza pan onto the grill and cook for 3 minutes until the cheese melts. Slice and serve your delicious cauliflower pizza.

Flatbreads Mediterranean

Prep Time: 10 min

Cook Time: 10 min

Serve: 6

Ingredients:

- 4 ounce marinated artichoke hearts
- 2 cups baby spinach
- 1/2 cup cherry tomatoes halved
- 2/3 cup cannellini beans
- 1/2 cup medium avocado sliced
- 1/4 cup cherry tomatoes halved
- 2 ounces crumbled feta cheese
- 1/4 small red onion peeled and sliced
- 1/4 cup almond

- 1/8 tsp ground black pepper
- 1tbsp olive oil
- 2 tbsp water
- 3 pieces of pita bread
- 1/4 tsp for slat some extra for sprinkling

Preparation:

1. Set your oven to 350 degrees F. At the same time pour beans into a food processor. Add your basil spinach salt pepper olive oil almonds and water together and pulse for 1 minute until smooth.

2. Place your flatbreads on a baking sheet and spread the bean pesto on flatbreads. Top this with your tomatoes avocado chopped artichokes and onion. Sprinkle with cheese. Place your flatbread into the oven and let bake for 10 minutes or until the pita bread is lightly crispy. When done cut each pizza in slices and serve.

Spinach Feta Grilled Cheese

Prep Time: 10 min

Cook Time: 18 min

Serve: 2

Ingredients:

- 1/4 pound spinach
- ½ teaspoon garlic
- 1/8 teaspoon salt
- 1/8 teaspoon ground black pepper
- 1/8 teaspoon red pepper flakes
- 1/2 tablespoons olive oil
- 1 cup shredded mozzarella cheese
- 2 tablespoons crumbled feta cheese
- 2 ciabatta rolls halved

Preparation:

1. Place a medium skillet pan over medium-low heat add oil and when hot add garlic. Cook for 2 minutes or until fragrant then add spinach and stir until mixed.

2. Turn heat to medium level and cook spinach for 5 minutes or until heated through and all the cooking liquid evaporates. Season with salt and black pepper and remove the pan from heat.

3. Spread ¼ cup of mozzarella cheese and 1 tablespoon feta cheese onto the bottom half of each roll top evenly with cooked spinach and then sprinkle with red pepper flakes.

4. Sprinkle with remaining mozzarella cheese and cover with top half of roll. Place a large skillet pan over medium heat and place sandwiches in it.

5. Fill a large pot half full with water and place on the sandwich to press them like Panini press. Switch heat

to medium-low level and cook for 5 minutes or until bottom is crispy. Then remove the pot flip the sandwich carefully top again with pot and continue cooking for another 5 minutes or until the other side is crispy and cheese melts completely.

6. Serve when ready.

Hummus

Prep/Cook time: 10 min

Serve: 16

Ingredients:

- 1 (14-ounce) can chickpeas drained
- 3 garlic cloves minced
- 2 tablespoons tallith
- 2 tablespoons extra-virgin olive oil
- Juice of 1 lemon
- Zest of 1 lemon
- 1/2 teaspoon sea salt
- Pinch cayenne pepper
- 2 tablespoons chopped fresh Italian parsley leaves

Preparation:

In a blender combine the chickpeas garlic tahini olive oil lemon juice and zest sea salt and cayenne. Blend for about 60 seconds until smooth. Garnish with parsley and serve.

Baba Ganoush(Vegan)

Prep Time: 10 min

Cook time: 15 min

Serve: 6

Ingredients:

- 1 eggplant peeled and sliced
- 1/4 cup tallini
- 1/2 teaspoon sea salt
- Juice of 1 lemon
- 1/4 teaspoon ground cumin
- 1/8 teaspoon freshly ground black pepper
- 2 tablespoons extra-virgin olive oil
- 2 tablespoons sunflower seeds (optional)
- 2 tablespoons fresh Italian

- parsley leaves (optional)

Preparation:

1. Preheat the oven to 350°F. Using a baking sheet spread the eggplant slices in an even layer. Bake for about 15 minutes until soft. Cool slightly and roughly chop the eggplant. In a blender blend the eggplant with the tahini sea salt lemon juice cumin and pepper for about 30 seconds. Transfer to a serving dish.

2. Drizzle with the olive oil and sprinkle with the sunflower seeds and parsley (if using) before serving.

Spiced Almonds

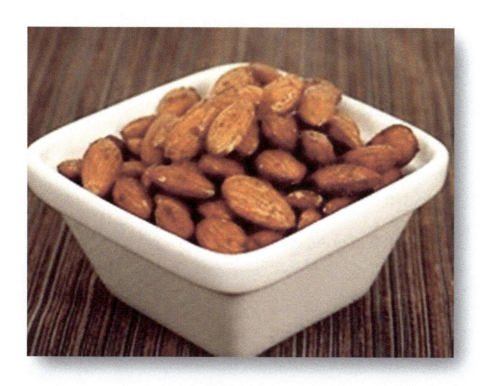

Prep Time: 10 min

Cook time: 7 min

Serve: 8

Ingredients:

- 2 cups raw unsalted almonds
- 1 tablespoon extra-virgin olive oil
- 1 teaspoon ground cumming
- 1/2 teaspoon garlic powder
- 1/2 teaspoon sea salt
- 1/8 teaspoon cayenne pepper

Preparation:

1. In a large nonstick skillet over medium-high heat cook the almonds for about 3 minutes shaking the pan constantly until the almonds become fragrant. Transfer to a bowl and set aside. In the same skillet over medium-high heat heat the olive oil until it shimmers.

2. Add the cumin garlic powder sea salt and cayenne. Cook for 30 to 60 seconds until the spices become fragrant.

3. Add the almonds to the skillet. Cook for about 3 minutes more stirring until the spices coat the almonds.

4. Let it cool before serving.

Lightning Source UK Ltd.
Milton Keynes UK
UKHW021822160421
382091UK00005B/51

9 781801 903004